Transforming Negative Core Beliefs Using Radical Imagination Therapy (RIT)

By

D. Trent Lewis MSW., LICSW

And

Laurel B. Damsel MSW., LICSW

This book is dedicated to the memory of Ron Klein, Founder and Director of the American Hypnosis Training Academy of Silver Spring, MD. His extraordinary teaching will be remembered for years to come and his influence will span future generations of psychotherapists.

"I had to clear up my idea that I was a worthless person. Because until I did, I acted like I was a worthless person. I did things that were self-destructive to confirm that I was a worthless person. I am so glad that I believe I am really OK." (D. Trent Lewis)

Forward

In many ways, negative core beliefs are in the eye of the beholder. They can be positive to some people and negative to others. Sometimes they can make perfect sense and other times they can defy reality altogether. Once they get established, however, they very often develop a life of their own and are perpetuated endlessly. They get encoded in the unconscious mind and some people will defend them to their very death. These beliefs are not only problematic for the persons harboring them, but for society as a whole. They are the cause of many of society's most pressing and destructive problems, such as racism, sexual exploitation, criminal activity, alcoholism, drug abuse, suicide, cults of all sorts, greed, poverty, authoritarianism, discrimination, and even war. Many of the people who harbor negative core beliefs do not see, nor will some ever see, that their core beliefs are a problem. Frequently, there are large payoffs for these people (i.e., money, status, power, control, sexual gratification, self-elevation, etc.). Just sometimes, however, there is a wake-up call, and they come to realize that their beliefs are not serving them well and are harmful to themselves or others. This wakeup call offers up a chance for change and a glimmer of hope. This change, however, is often not an easy process, but it can and does happen.

In the best of all worlds, negative core beliefs would never get started in the first place. They would be prevented. Positive parenting and education aimed at ethical responsibility and social inclusiveness would go a long way in doing this. Currently, we are far from this ideal.

Once negative core beliefs take hold, there is the problem of how to best deal with them. I will always remember what Steve Andreas once said in a Psychotherapy Networker workshop: "Symptoms don't like to be erased or eliminated. They get pissed." (Steve Andreas). That statement is also so true for negative core beliefs. Instead, they require a transformation. That transformation can come in many different forms (i.e., a personal awakening related to harm being done to the self or others; new learning or education, positive or negative reinforcement, effective laws and legislation, etc.). In this book, we are proposing another solution: Radical Imagination Therapy, or RIT. We believe it to be an effective and innovative way of dealing with this very perplexing and difficult problem which affects so many people.

Acknowledgements

We have many people to thank related to the concepts and ideas presented in this book which deal with Negative Core Beliefs and Radical Imagination Therapy (RIT). First and foremost, we would like to thank the late Ron Klein, Director and Founder of the American Hypnosis Training Academy, whose excellent training workshops introduced us to many of the techniques and concepts found in this publication. Ron was truly an innovative educator ahead of his time. Others who we have mentioned in our previous publications include: Milton H. Erickson, Virginia Satir, Jeffrey Zeig, Ernest Rossie, Jay Haley, Richard Bandler, John Grinder, Robert Dilts, Judith Delozer, Stephen Gilligan, Michael Yapko, Michelle Weine Davis, Steve deShazer, Steve Andreas, Richard Simon, Francine Shapiro and Albert Pessio. All of these people have made major contributions to our thinking which relate to the transformation of negative core beliefs. There are of course many others who we give our thanks and gratitude to as well.

Our usual thank you goes out to Mrs. Susan Weidner, Dr. Robert Weidner, my son Matthew Lewis, his wife Katie Lewis, my daughter Jenny Lewis, Duina Reyes, for back cover photos and my loving wife and co-author Laurel Damsel. To everyone, we give a big heartfelt thank you.

Introduction

Almost everyone has heard the question: "Do you think that you have bit off a little more than you can chew?" In dealing with the topic of transforming negative core beliefs, I say maybe we have, but for any of us to move forward in life, we need to push the limits and tackle the hard problems in order to come up with better and more positive solutions. Transforming negative core beliefs is no exception. Before beginning the transformation process, we need to first define core beliefs and their characteristics. Core beliefs can best be defined as well-established and ingrained patterns of thoughts and behaviors that are of significant importance to an individual or group of individuals. They must also have payoffs, which in some way meets a particular need or needs for those individuals. Certainly, there are both positive and negative core beliefs and we would hazard to guess that most core beliefs are positive. Negative core beliefs, on the other hand, are those beliefs which are in some way harmful to the self or to others. In contrasting positive and negative core beliefs, one could say that positive core beliefs can be very useful to people and to society. The direct opposite is true of negative core beliefs. A few examples of positive core beliefs include: being helpful to others, kindness, honesty, truthfulness, generosity, inclusiveness, positive regard for others, etc. In other words, they follow the "Golden Rule" which states: "Do unto others as you would have others do unto you."

In considering both positive and negative core beliefs, we need to take a long look at the payoffs involved. Payoffs are always there. In order for any change to occur, there needs to be stronger and more powerful payoffs than the ones keeping the negative beliefs in place. Although changing negative core beliefs can be difficult, it is certainly not impossible. Quality education is a great way to do this as well as preventing them from getting started in the first place. Teaching children from an early age to respect themselves as well as others makes a big difference.

In this book, we will be focusing on using imagination as a pathway for change. We have identified four steps in this process. The first and most difficult step is that of acceptance. This step is difficult in that it requires admitting there is a problem in the first place and a need to change it. It is kind of like the alcoholic admitting out loud in an AA meeting: "My name is Joe and I am an alcoholic." That is often the hardest obstacle to get over. The second step for change is that of planning. This step is wide open for all sorts of innovative ideas and techniques which require imagination and individualization. That is to say, in the planning process, one needs to incorporate what had been learned about the person and utilize it for positive change. Interests, strengths, and abilities can be incorporated here. The third step in the process is implementation. This step requires a commitment on the part of the individual to follow a mutually agreed on plan. This step also requires a solid contract to carry out the plan. Milton Erickson would often insist on this with his clients. The fourth and final step is repetition and more repetition. Repetition helps to establish and solidify those new and better neuro-networks aiding in the change process. In this final step, it is also helpful to chart one's progress. We have suggested a one to ten rating scale with one being the most progress and ten being the least. Here we chart the progress toward the goal of transformational change (See Appendix #7). Before getting into our examples of transforming negative core beliefs, let us first begin by providing a brief review of Radical Imagination Therapy (RIT).

What is Radical Imagination Therapy?

For our readers unfamiliar with Radical Imagination Therapy or RIT, we would like to give you some background information on it. There is a very good synopsis of it in our first book, The Principles and Methods of Radical Imagination Therapy (D. Trent Lewis and Laurel B. Damsel). In a nutshell, Radical Imagination Therapy is a form of therapy that utilizes imagination to change the perception of a problematic issue. It is very imaginative and creative in the techniques which are employed and really, the sky is the limit when using it. We do things such as create and act out imaginary scenarios with solutions imbedded in them. We put great emphasis on emotion and exaggeration using hand gestures, facial expressions, voice tone, changing size, and many other things. We can use angels, fairies, spiritual guides, wizards, and helpers of all sorts. We may use colored balls of healing light that we toss around. We may stand up or walk through a problem. We may change the distance, color, sound, or feel of a problem. We often use humor, sing songs, or do ridiculous things such as making our big toe talk or sing to us (Steve Andreas). We may also use nonsense language to break into the dysfunctional thought patterns (i.e., Blah, Blah, Blah or Da, Da, Da). (D. Trent Lewis, Laurel B. Damsel). These techniques are formulated to alter the way a problem is perceived in order to consolidate a new and better memory for healing purposes. In order to reinforce this process of change, we encourage the use of meditation. We utilize a quick five second meditation technique to make this process simple (Appendix #1).

Radical Imagination Therapy is, as the name suggests, meant to be radical. It breaks into the negative loops of our thought processes and stimulates the mind in ways that makes it possible for new and better thinking and behavior to occur. The human mind has plasticity and that plasticity can be used for positive change. There was a great bumper sticker in one of my previous offices which said, "Subvert the Dominant Paradigm." I felt that it was so true that when a dominant paradigm was negative or dysfunctional, it needed to be subverted. What better way to subvert it than to radically alter it in some way. My new bumper sticker would read, "Transform the Negative Paradigm." Although similar, this message better captures what we are doing when using RIT. We are altering the negative core belief and doing it in a very powerful and creative way.

Milton Erickson was a master at observation, creativity, and individualization. For RIT to work well, it needs to hit the mark. Careful observation needs to be done regarding the problem and the unique nature of the person or persons requiring change. Each person is a unique individual and the therapy utilized needs be adapted to the specific needs of that individual. (Milton H. Erickson) Just the right recipe needs to be formulated to make the change required. Because RIT is so creative and flexible, it is well suited to do just that.

The Four Stages of Transformation

The four stages of transformation related to changing negative core beliefs using RIT are: acceptance, planning, implementation, and repetition. As stated earlier, some people will never come to the point of wanting to change their negative core beliefs. Their pay offs are just too great. However, for those people who do wish to make changes, RIT offers them very creative and effective ways to do so.

Acceptance

The first stage of transformation is acceptance and, as stated earlier, it is by far the hardest to overcome. People will hold onto core beliefs with all their might until something either positive or negative challenges the payoffs that they are getting from them. One of the biggest motivators for people to change is the realization that their negative core beliefs are so harmful to themselves or others that change is necessary. People caught up in cults or bullying can and do experience this. For example, a bully may see the devastating effects that their bullying has on their innocent victims. Intervention may not be necessary in such cases. On the other hand, an RIT therapist may be useful in helping the bully to see the positive payoffs that they can get from not doing the behavior.

Planning

The second stage of transforming negative core beliefs is planning. In order to plan a change, the therapist must have a good understanding of the individual and their needs. Utilizing RIT is like fitting the right puzzle piece into the puzzle. It requires coming up with just the right technique to use for that particular individual (Milton H. Erickson). Observation and personal history are key. The therapist needs to know as much as they can about the person (i.e., likes and dislikes, interests, learning style, cultural influences, favorite stories, hobbies, modes of socialization, etc.). The therapist can utilize this information to assist the client in planning a transformation. There also must be a willingness on the part of the individual to try something different and very much out of the ordinary. They must be educated related to thinking about and doing things which may seem very strange and even ridiculous to them. Usually, however, this can be fairly easy to overcome by educating them on the radical nature of the therapy and how it can help them with their problem. Our best way to explain this process is by giving some examples and illustrations which will follow later in this book.

Implementation

After careful planning and choosing the right technique, the third step is implementation. Often, Milton Erickson would use explicit directives and encourage his clients to follow them exactly as he prescribed. Because he was known to be such a renowned physician and therapist, they would do so and were often amazed at the changes they had made. The therapist using RIT techniques can learn much from his approach. After all, the goal for clients is the resolution of their problems; following explicit directives should be stressed as a way to do this.

Repetition

The fourth and final step of transformation is that of repetition. It is important that the implementation process be continually reinforced until it becomes habitual. Like anything else that we do, being persistent is the key here. By doing things over and over, it becomes so ingrained that it is almost like tying your shoes. There is an old saying that to really master something you must do it at least ten thousand times. This concept was brought out in a hypnosis training workshop given by the late Ron Klein at the American Hypnosis Training Academy. This may be just a little overstated, but I tend to agree with him that only by doing something over and over again repeatedly is one able to really become proficient at it. Transforming negative core beliefs is no different. It takes work.

Let's now get into the nitty gritty of the transformation process by providing some illustrations starting with self-destructive self-talk.

Negative Self Talk

A few years before his death, Steve Andreas wrote a book which was titled *Transforming Negative Self-Talk: Practical Effective Exercises* (Steve Andreas). In this book, he talked a great deal about really looking at the validity of what the person was saying to themselves. Was what was being said internally really true in all respects? Many times, by looking at this negative self-talk in a systematic way, the person sees how illogical it really is. Sometimes when analyzing it, it may even seem ridiculous to the person. At a Psychotherapy Networker Symposium workshop, he demonstrated this in a very humorous way by advising a person with negative self-talk to have their big toe sing a song about how terrible they were and then hearing a different song in the background sung by their little toe with a more positive affirmation about themselves. It completely changed their perception of the negative self-talk by demonstrating how ridiculous and illogical the first song was and how self-affirming the second one seemed to be (Steve Andreas). Let's now give a couple of illustrations of how negative self-talk can be transformed using our fictional characters of Joe and Joleen.

Illustration #1

Joleen was raised in a very dysfunctional household. Her father was alcoholic and abusive and her mother was very codependent and passive. Joleen was the oldest of five children and took it upon herself to be the responsible one for the family. In fact, even her mother would often ask her for advice at a very early age when she was ill-equipped to give it. The family was very poor and often had to depend on food stamps in order to have enough to eat. Joleen did her best to make sure her siblings didn't go without the food and care that they needed. She was very much admired by everyone, however, she paid a dear price for that adulation. Joleen would often question herself and blame herself if for some reason something in the family didn't work out. She always felt that it was her responsibility and her fault. She developed what might be termed as the "it's my fault syndrome." This became so internalized that even when the slightest thing went wrong, she would say to herself: "That was my fault."

 Despite all of the family dysfunction, Joleen did quite well in school and was very well-liked by other students and teachers. She did her best to please all of the other people around her, however, she paid a big price for all of her diligence. She felt like she could never be wrong and always felt on edge. As time went on and she grew to be young a young woman, Joleen kept on trying to please everyone. For the most part she was successful, however, she never felt worthy. She would sometimes say to herself that she wished she never was born and that the world would be better off without her. Despite this, Joleen went on to graduate from high school got a job working as an administrative assistant for a small construction company. There she met her husband and soon became pregnant with her first child. It was at that time that things got worse for her and she fell into a serious depression and became suicidal. Her doctor referred her to a therapist connected to her practice. At first, it was thought that she might have postpartum depression and her symptoms were severe enough to require hospitalization. It was there that she attended groups and was placed on medication. In learning more about Joleen's history, her therapist decided to recommend RIT to deal with her negative self-talk. Her therapist learned that Joleen loved ballet dancing and while growing up she would often practice ballet on her own even though her family could not afford to send her to any classes. Along with the usual individual and group therapy in the hospital, Joleen was taught how to meditate and it was suggested that she meditate on being a magnificent ballerina dancing in front of a large audience. It was further suggested that she give her meditation details, with wonderful colors, costumes and audience adulation. Her therapist suggested that whenever she would have any sort of negative self-talk that she would bring the vision of this meditation into her mind. She further reinforced it by giving her the suggestion that she touch her fore finger and thumb together. Any time she would talk in a negative way about herself she should do this. This is called a "power anchor," which brings to mind her perception of herself as a wonderful and talented ballerina in a tactile way. Also, because Joleen loved to use her iPhone, her therapist suggested that she come up with a positive affirmation about herself that she could agree with and put it on an automatic alert which would go off every 6 hours. Joleen came up with a statement: "I am OK just the way I am, despite not being perfect." It was suggested that she devise other positive affirmations and put them on her phone as well.

Almost immediately after using these techniques for only a few days, Joleen began to notice a very positive difference in the way she felt about herself. She was delighted. A few months later, she was inspired to seek out and join an adult ballet class. This further reinforced her new born positive feelings about herself.

Great care should be taken to make the imagined visualizations and auditory messages as powerful as possible. This helps for these solutions to stick and be encoded in the brain. Doing such things as adding colors, making things bigger, zooming in and out, making the sounds louder or softer all aid in this process. Even changing the timelines to past present and future make a difference in our perception. (Steve Andreas) Our brains have neuroplasticity and all of these processes help to encode the new and better solution.

Illustration #2

Our next case illustration involves Joe, who was bullied as a child while growing up. Unfortunately, Joe was born with a cleft lip and palate and although he had an operation to repair them, he was left with a slight scar and speech impediment. While growing up, other children picked up on these deformities and called him names. Joe never felt like he belonged, and except for a very few close friends he felt a sense of rejection by others. Joe knew he was different and would come down on himself with some very negative internal dialog. He would think and say to himself such things as: "I'm no good for nothing;" and "I'm nothing but a freak to look at." Joe stayed to himself a lot and would not put himself into situations where he would be noticed. Joe had many talents and where he really excelled was running. Joe was by far the fastest runner in his school and was asked to join the track team. His specialty was the 100 meter dash and in the state finals he took first place. Despite his great achievements, Joe held onto his negative feelings about his looks and his speech. Although many people had great admiration for Joe and his accomplishments, he continued to hold onto his negative feelings about himself and his negative self-talk. His track coach noted how depressed and unhappy he seemed and recommended that he see a counselor. Joe agreed and he went in for a mental health assessment at a clinic in his neighborhood. Joe was fortunate to get a counselor familiar with problems like his and recommended (CBT Cognitive Behavioral Therapy) combined with Radical Imagination Therapy (RIT). His therapist decided to be very creative in his use of RIT. Because he knew that Joe was a negative self- talker and that a change of perception was necessary, he decided to use humor as a way to help Joe change the way he perceived himself. He knew that it would be very important for the humor to be used in a way that would not be at all mocking of Joe, so he prepared him that the techniques that he would be using would seem very strange and unusual and that in no way did he want to offend him. Joe was very curious about this approach, so he agreed to give this therapy a try.

His therapist asked Joe what type of humorous animal he would be if that were possible. Joe said that he often felt like an ugly duckling. That was not the response his therapist would like to have heard, however, he decided to use it anyway to assist Joe in making up a healing story. His therapist asked Joe to think of that ugly duckling doing something funny or heroic that was of benefit to others. Joe said it was hard but that he would try to come up with something. There wasn't time for Joe to think of a story on the spot, so his therapist advised him to come in with his story at his next therapy appointment.

When he arrived, Joe presented the following positive story about the ugly duckling: "Once upon a time there was a strange looking ugly duckling, very different than the other ducklings which were hatched. He was truly a sight to see, with large webbed feet and a long neck. Because of his long neck, he couldn't quack like the other ducklings. He made a strange sound when he tried and felt very much out of place. As time went on, he felt more and more like a freak and would mostly just stay to himself away from the other ducks. He was, however, a great swimmer and diver because of his feet, and would often catch the biggest fish in the pond. The other ducks would admire him for that but he still felt like he was strange and out of place. He would constantly say to himself, 'I am a freak!' One summer, however, everything changed for him when the weather got very hot and all the fish went to the bottom of the pond in order to survive. The other ducks were unable to dive deep enough to get any fish except for him. The entire

group of ducks began to starve as the heat destroyed
their food supply. Seeing their terrible situation, the ugly
duckling dove deep to the bottom of the pond and
brought fish to the other ducks. He became their hero
and saved their lives. That ugly duckling never felt like
he was a freak again and the other ducks included him in
all of their activities."

His therapist really liked Joe's imaginary story and
encouraged him to meditate on it each night before he
went to bed. He advised him to add color, sound, and
feeling to the story each time he visualized it to
strengthen the memory. He also advised Joe to keep
track of how he felt and how often he would get the
negative self-talk. He did this in a notebook. To his
surprise and delight, Joe reported feeling much improved
over just a couple of weeks. He said that he felt that
being a little different wasn't all that bad after all. His
coach also noted a big difference in Joe's confidence
level and mood.

Eating Disorders

Eating disorders are very common and also very debilitating. One of the most common is binge eating and purging (bulimia). According to statistics from NIH, the lifetime prevalence of binge eating and purging (bulima) is 2. 8% in the U.S. Although less common, another major eating disorder is that of anorexia nervosa. The lifetime prevalence of anorexia nervosa is 0.6%.with women being the most affected (three times higher than men). We also have a very serious obsity problem in this country. It is estimated that in the United States over 70 million people are obese (Wikipedia). Along with poor food choices, people overeat or under-eat for many different reasons. Negative core beliefs often play a large role here. These beliefs can get installed for a wide variety of reasons and are often very difficult to control. The first step, of course, is to recognize the problem and the need for change. For those people who get past this first step, there is reason for hope. We feel that RIT can be a very powerful tool in helping people to move beyond the negative core beliefs that drive these eating disorders. Our next two illustrations demonstrate this.

Illustration #3

Joleen is a 24 year old college student with a long history of binge eating and purging which first started in high school. Like many others with this problem, she did it in secret. Joleen was teased as a child because of her weight and often called "a fatty" by her schoolmates. Her mother didn't help this situation by being critical of her eating habits and how she looked. This entire situation set Joleen up for her bulimia. She found that through purging she was able to come down to a normal weight range, however, this was done at a terrible price. She found herself pale and sickly with frequent bouts of gastric and dental problems. Despite these problems, for years, she kept her secret hidden from others as a result of shame and embarrassment.

When she entered college her problems worsened. At one point, Joleen found that she was so sick that she could not go to class. Finally, she did go to the campus health center where she admitted her problem to the doctor. After a full diagnostic workup, she was referred for counseling. Her therapist was familiar with bulimia and had treated a number of other students with this problem. She soon discovered that Joleen, like many others, had a core belief that being overweight was one of the worst things that could happen to anyone. She was in a negative self-perpetuating loop which kept her on this path of destruction. She knew that treating Joleen's long standing problem with bulimia would not be easy, however, having successfully used both Radical Imagination Therapy and Cognitive Behavioral Therapy before, recovery is possible.

One of the important things that her therapist learned from her evaluation was that Joleen loved animals and she had a cat named Fluffy, who would often sleep with her at night on her bed. She would sometimes hold Fluffy and cuddle with her. Knowing from experience that in order to change a problem, a person needs to do something different as it relates to the problem, she decided to give Joleen a directive which would help her to perceive her problem in a different way utilizing her cat Fluffy. The first thing that she did was to instruct Joleen on how to meditate using the five second breathing technique (Appendix #1). Next, during her meditation, she advised Joleen to think about cuddling with Fluffy. As she was doing this, it was suggested that she put her hand over her heart and visualize this experience including all of the feelings and sounds associated with it (i.e., cat purring, the feeling of her fur, etc.). During her daily activities, she was also encouraged to put her hand over her heart (power anchor) whenever her she had the desire to binge and purge. She was also given the homework assignment of charting her progress. Her therapist knew from experience that there may be setbacks, however, when they would happen, she was encouraged to never give up and stay on track. She was advised to reinforce this process with increased periods of meditation and the hand over heart technique. She explained to Joleen that relapses are to be expected, however, they can be overcome with persistence and perseverance.

Joleen made very good progress using this simple form of therapy. Within just two weeks she had only one relapse and was able to get back on track almost immediately. She felt that with the use of both Cognitive Behavioral Therapy and Radical Imagination Therapy, she saw a bright future for herself without bulimia.

Next, let us move on to anorexia nervosa. Most treatment specialists would agree that in order to deal with it most effectively, it requires a team approach. Much like bulimia, very often negative core beliefs play a major role in its development and continuation. In order to treat it most effectively, a change in how they perceive themselves is required. Most see themselves as being fat or overweight even though the opposite is clearly the case. We are convinced that Radical Imagination Therapy combined with other treatment modalities, can effectively be a way to make this happen. Our next illustration demonstrates this process.

Illustration #4

Joe is a 25 year old openly gay young man who has had anorexia since his mid-teens. Joe had a very difficult time accepting his sexuality during his formative years and only very recently shared with his family, friends, and relatives that he was gay. Joe was always thin as a child and for the most part, other people in his life did not pay much attention to his thin stature. Like many others with anorexia, Joe had a distorted image of himself as being heavy and overweight even though the opposite was true. He felt like he needed to eat less in order to look his best. Even though his eating disorder was never addressed, he was able to finish high school as well as college. His major in college was graphic design and he was extraordinarily talented at it. He was hired immediately after earning his degree by a large advertising company. It was at that time that he entered into a relationship which only lasted for a couple of months. Joe blamed himself for the breakup. This stress, along with his perfectionism at work caused Joe to literally starve himself. He became so under nourished that one day he fainted at his desk. His supervisor called for an ambulance and he was taken to the emergency room of a local hospital.

The doctor in the emergency room took one look at Joe and saw that he required admission. After a complete workup, a diagnosis of anorexia nervosa was made and when he was ready for discharge, he was referred for nutritional support as well as psychological therapy. The therapist that he was referred to was very skilled in both CBT and RIT. In learning about Joe's talents in graphic design, his therapist suggested that he use a technique whereby Joe would create an imaginary healing story using his graphic design skills. He was given an assignment to create a character with a problem similar to his own and in graphics, create a very radical and unique positive solution to it. Joe was very inspired by this assignment and he came up with an idea of creating a Healing Temple, where people would go to be healed from all sorts of ailments. It was a magnificent creation, not only on the outside but on the inside as well. It was elegantly furnished with tapestry, an internal golden archway, jewels, and crystals. When someone came in needing healing, they would pass through the golden archway into a room which was lighted by all the colors of the rainbow. They would be engulfed in a radiant light and be instantly healed, looking healthy and robust at an ideal weight - not too thin and not too heavy. Joe's therapist instructed him to draw this out in graphic form and then meditate on it using the five second breathing technique of meditation (Appendix #1). This was his homework assignment, as well as charting his progress on a one to ten scale (Appendix #7).

This assignment proved to be a game changer for Joe. When he came in for his next appointment, he looked better physically and reported that he was feeling better emotionally as well. He was giving himself ones and twos on the rating scale, which, to Joe, was amazing. His therapist advised him to continue doing what he was doing, including repeating his visualizations over and over (repetition).

Why did this technique work so well? I feel strongly that it was because Joe came up with the idea himself with just a little guidance from his therapist. Also, his ability and talent in graphic design played a significant part here. He was able to draw out his solution in detail using his excellent skills and abilities. Milton Erickson would be very pleased in how keen observation and utilization contributed to Joe's healing (Milton H. Erickson).

Addictions

Next, let us move on to addictions as they relate to RIT transforming negative core beliefs. When speaking about addictions, usually there are very valid reasons for them. These reasons can be very complex, and treating them can be very complex as well. Alcohol and drugs are by far the most common addictions and often require specialized treatment. As a result of their physical effects on the body, detoxification and medications are often utilized as the first steps in this process. Because we are dealing here with the psychological issues related to negative core beliefs, we will quickly move beyond the initial detoxification process.

Illustration #5

Let's begin with Joe, a 24 year old young adult, who has been addicted to a wide variety of drugs for the past 5 years. Joe came from a very dysfunctional family. His father was an alcoholic and his mother very codependent. Joe's father was described as being very abusive when intoxicated and would often take his anger out on Joe and his mother. His father would hit his mother and often rage at Joe and saying things like: "You are nothing but a little wimp and will never amount to anything." That was something Joe never forgot and was also what he began thinking about himself. He became a troubled child, getting into fights at school and hanging around other kids who acted out in a similar way. Soon he got into alcohol and began abusing nearly every drug that was available. Early on in his addiction, he would break into houses with his friends and steal things to support his alcohol and drug abuse. Later, he began selling drugs to other addicts. He was caught several times by the police and because he was a minor at the time he was placed on probation for his offenses. This did not deter Joe and he continued in his criminal ways. He was locked up for a few months during these years but when he was caught selling large quantities of opiates he was given a 2 year mandatory sentence. It was at this time that he met a prison counselor who felt that Joe might be responsive to RIT. In doing his assessment, he learned about Joe's early childhood experiences and about his core belief that he would never amount to anything. He felt that this core belief set him up for a life of failure. He asked Joe if he would be willing to try out RIT therapy. Joe thought it was a little weird, however, he agreed to give it a try.

Joe's therapist explained the process of RIT to him and taught him how to meditate using the five second countdown technique (Appendix #1). During his assessment, he learned that Joe loved to make pizza, especially the crust. At that time, Joe was working in the kitchen where he was involved in baking all sorts of meals, including pizza. His therapist decided to incorporate Joe's interest and abilities in baking with the RIT therapy. Using his imagination, he asked Joe to project himself into the future and create a "best case scenario" for himself related to pizza making. He advised him to make up a success based story related to his pizza making. He was further advised to make the story full of all sorts of amazing and vivid images. Joe thought this was a strange, but because it was described as being Radical Imagination Therapy he decided to play along. At his next therapy session he came up with the idea that in the distant future he would own chain of pizza parlors called "Crusty Joe's Pizzas." He said that each pizza parlor would have a signature sign with very colorful lights around it. He said he saw cars lined up to pick up their pizza and people inside enjoying his crusty delicious pizza. Joe's therapist very much liked his vision and encouraged him to make it as vivid as he could describing it in the smallest detail (i.e., customers coming in, smiles on their faces, happy employees, ovens fully loaded with crusty pizzas, etc.). He then encouraged Joe to meditate on this vision each night before going to sleep in his prison bunk bed.

Joe did this dutifully and during his next session reported back that it was actually fun to do this meditation. His therapist encouraged Joe to continue to modify his imagined scenario, doing such things as visualizing all sorts of people eating his pizza, changing the time line as how his chain of pizza parlors grew from the past to the present and into the future. (Steve Andreas) Joe picked up on these suggestions well and reported back that he was able to create an amazing variety of imaginary stories regarding his pizza business that it was very pleasant to meditate on. His positive stories were always changing and very dynamic.

As the months went by, Joe began to think differently about himself. That old core belief that he was just "a little wimp and that he would never amount to anything" began to fade. He even began to become more confident about trying out new pizza baking ideas in the prison kitchen. Joe gradually came to believe that he could become a different and more positive person. We will let our readers imagine on their own how his use of RIT turned out when he was released from prison.

Addictions come in many different forms, as do their solutions. Joe's is only one example. RIT seeks to find just the right recipe for each one. Some of the techniques utilized include imaginary stories, the miracle question, modifying real life scenarios, the use of spiritual helpers, famous figures of all sorts, even the use of crystals or religious artifacts. The recipes and techniques are limitless. Individualization is the key and it has to be something that is strong enough to overpower the compulsion to indulge (Appendix#2).

Hoarding

Hoarding is a big problem for many people and it deserves some attention here related to negative core beliefs. When talking about hoarding, you are also taking about an addiction and a compulsion. It too has its own etiology and reasons for self-perpetuating. According to Wikipedia, the overall incidence of compulsive hoarding is 2.6% with higher rates of those over 60 years of age and people with other psychiatric diagnoses, especially anxiety and depression. (Wikipedia) It is a debilitating disorder that can and does destroy lives. Like other addictions and compulsions, hoarding can manifest in many different forms. It can be specific to hoarding one particular item or multiple items. Each person is unique and should be treated as such. The following case illustration demonstrates how RIT has been able to help people with this serious problem.

Illustration #6

Joleen, age 45, is a medically disabled police officer who was seriously injured when a routine traffic stop went bad. While standing beside the road, she was hit by a speeding car, which resulted in a severe concussion and major injuries to her legs. Unable to perform her duties, she was retired on permanent medical disability. It was shortly after her retirement that Joleen began to fill her house with all sorts of items (i.e., food, clothes, newspapers, things she saw at stores, etc.). She found it hard to part with anything she was attracted to and whenever her two adult children came over to visit, they were appalled at what they saw. Her hoarding was at a point where it was hard to get in and out of her house and became a health hazard. At first Joleen refused to admit that she had a problem, however, when the health department was called in and she was given an ultimatum to either clean up or have her home condemned that she finally made a decision to seek help. At the urging of her children, she agreed to see a therapist familiar with obsessive compulsive behaviors and hoarding.

During her first session, her therapist did a very thorough psychological assessment of Joleen. She learned that from a very early age, Joleen had to deal with deprivation. She was the oldest of three children raised by a single mother. Joleen's father died in a car accident when she was only seven years old. Her mother had to depend on a small Social Security check, public assistance and food pantries to get by during her early years. Joleen did all she could to help her mother care for her two younger sisters. The food assistance that the family received only helped somewhat to feed the family and the clothes that they wore had to come from thrift stores. During these early years, her mother was only able to get part time job caring for an elderly lady. Despite these hardships, Joleen and her sisters went on to finish high school. Joleen became interested in law enforcement and at that particular time they were looking for female recruits. She finished her training and became a police offer at the early age of 19. She soon married another police officer and had two children within three years. Her marriage ended in divorce and she assumed primary custody of her children. Accustomed to caregiving, she was able to manage her job responsibilities as well as those of being a single mother. As time marched on, her children grew up and they assumed lives on their own. It was just after her younger daughter's wedding that her accident happened. The accident and subsequent disability retirement seemed to be the tipping point for Joleen. She started buying things that she didn't need or use. When her two daughters moved out on their own she no longer had anyone to care for and no longer felt a need to keep her house organized and in order. Within just a few short months things began to spiral out of control. Very soon her house became overloaded with things she didn't need or use. She even saved newspapers, which she stacked up in piles all over the house. Her hoarding problem literally buried her in items she thought to be indispensable but soon became a toxic pile of trash.

 Recalling Joleen's desire to help and care for others, her therapist decided to utilize this as a way to help her to gain control of her obsessive hoarding. She advised Joleen to imagine in her "mind's eye" how she might help someone with a hoarding problem similar to her own. This was her first homework assignment. She was taught how to meditate using the five second breathing technique (Appendix #1) and was instructed to meditate on how she would be helpful to such a person each night before her bedtime. She was further instructed to make her meditations as visual and real as possible giving them a color, a feel, and even sounds. Although Joleen was very skeptical at first, she carried out these instructions to the letter. Also, because of the possible condemnation of her property, she was referred to a cleaning company which had experience with hoarding behavior. Within just two short weeks, Joleen began to show amazing progress. She reported being able to clean out the newspapers and to make donations of clothing and other items that she no longer needed. She said that the meditations related to helping a person with her same problem made all the difference. Joleen found herself well on the way to recovery. Her therapist also referred her to a hoarders support group which she willingly joined. She felt that by assisting Joleen to get in touch with her care giving needs, she would ultimately be able to help herself to recover.

Not all hoarding behaviors are as easy to modify as Joleen's. However, by individualizing the therapy and utilizing their positive strengths, good results can be achieved. In Joleen's case, her core belief was that of deprivation and there never being enough. Each person's situation is different and the treatment approach requires that it be tailored to those individual differences (Milton H. Erickson).

Cults

Next, let us consider cults as they relate to negative core beliefs. A huge amount of information is available on cults in books, articles, TV documentaries and studies of all sorts. As an example, just take look at Wikipedia under cults. This only scratches the surface on the topic. Much of this information relates to the great harm done by cults and deservingly so.

So what is a cult and how does it relate to negative core beliefs? I would hazard to say that there is no simple answer to this question. In defining a cult, one could say that it is an ideology which is accepted and followed by an individual or group of individuals which in some way meets their particular needs. How this ideology is viewed is a matter for one's interpretation. Cults usually have a charismatic leader or even a group of leaders who profess the ideology. Cults in and of themselves may not be bad - unless they take advantage of others or do harm in some way to others which includes the members themselves. Cults are tricky in that they can appear to do good things, however, they can be very destructive in that they have the capacity to limit or take away a person's free will. Charismatic cult leaders are often very narcissistic and domineering. They can very easily exploit others related to their freedom of choice in order to meet the cult leaders' needs, whatever they may be (i.e., power, money, sexual gratification etc.). Exploitation is a common theme.

Breaking away from a cult can be very difficult for many people because of the strong indoctrination process and the beliefs which have been instilled in them. Once established, these beliefs tend to become core beliefs and are self-perpetuating. Believers themselves can reinforce the ideology within their own minds and many are drawn to try to indoctrinate and recruit others. Another problem related to breaking free is the bonding that takes place among cult members. There is a sense of belonging and often strong alliances and friendships develop between cult members. Leaving a cult means breaking free from these bonds, which can create feelings of loss, guilt, and even remorse. These reasons are often why cult members stay for as long as they do.

When a person does decide to leave a cult, there is almost always an overpowering reason for doing so. Sometimes the ideology just no longer makes sense to them. Other people leave because they have been mistreated in some way or see others who they have high regard for mistreated. This can be physical abuse, sexual abuse, emotional abuse or a number of other reasons. There are some people will never leave a cult for any reason. The bonds that are established in the cult are just too strong.

For those individuals who do decide to leave a cult, there is hope and help out there. There are a variety of paths one can take for healing. Certainly, individual and group support can be very helpful. Seeking out others who have left and mentally and emotionally processing the experience have assisted a great number of people to break free. Belonging to a cult and then leaving it is a life changing experience, never to be forgotten. The path one takes toward healing is an individual one. We are suggesting that RIT is only one of many possible ways to do this. The following illustration demonstrates the use of RIT in this process.

Illustration #7

Joe is a 26 year old man who has been involved in a religious cult for over 9 years. Like many others who join a cult, he was drawn in by a very charismatic and seductive leader. Joe was raised in a very religious family, and while growing up was a quite devoted member of a traditional Protestant church which he attended regularly with his family. It was only when Joe went off to college that he decided to explore other churches and religious alternatives. He had a college roommate who was attending religious services at a very nonconventional evangelistic church which sponsored frequent retreats at a country estate owned by one of the church members. The minister of the church claimed that he was chosen by God as a leader of this ministry, and that his spoken words came directly from God speaking through him. He was extremely charismatic and convincing and his enticing demeanor was very persuasive. Joe took to the church almost immediately and he became a very devoted member of the congregation. The minister required that his followers be obedient to God and because he professed to be one of God's chosen leaders, his followers were required to be obedient to him as well. Members were obligated to work for the church and give at least 50% of their income to the ministry. Members of the congregation were so devoted to this charismatic leader that they willingly did so. Members were also required to recruit others to the ministry as well. Joe eagerly followed these directives and he soon became a favored church member. As the church grew, so did its finances. The minister started using church resources to buy property and rent it out. Within just a few short years, the value of these properties was in the millions. The minister lived in a large mansion which was owned by the church. He had several expensive luxury cars which were also owned by the church. All of his entitlements were said to be God's will for him.

As time progressed, Joe noted that the minister's behavior became increasingly controlling and dictatorial. This was a gradual process which was largely ignored by the other church members. Joe noted that he began to require that women in the church dress in certain way and be compliant to his requests. Because they felt that these directives were from God, they willingly complied. Joe became concerned when one of the young women who he knew very well informed him that she was often asked to give massages to the minister and even perform sexual favors for him. Joe was so shocked and enraged when he learned about this that he felt that he could no longer be a part of this ministry. It was at that time that he decided to leave the congregation. This was very difficult for him in that he was so invested in the church and bonded to the other church members. His abrupt departure caused a big uproar among his close friends in the congregation. When they asked him why he was leaving, he told them that it was for some serious family problems which came up suddenly. He felt that he could not betray the confidence of his close female friend who confided in him. He felt very guilty about not sharing the whole truth but he found that he could no longer tolerate being a part of this ministry. As a result of this situation, Joe was shaken to his very core and became so anxious and depressed that he decided to seek professional help. He knew of a skilled pastoral counselor who he trusted and made an appointment as soon as he could.

Hearing Joe's story, his therapist knew right away that he was dealing with a religious cult and a very exploitative cult leader. Because Joe had been so bonded to this ministry, he knew that fully breaking free from the church would be extremely difficult. His primary bond was to the other church members who were as devoted as he once was. In considering Joe's dilemma, his therapist decided to use an RIT approach which involved imagining an ideal ministry which would never be exploitative or harmful in any way. This approach seemed a little strange to Joe, however, he had many very good ideas about what an ideal ministry would be like. Joe told his therapist that an ideal ministry would put God in charge, not any one person. The minister would be more of a shepherd and guide than an authoritarian leader. He said that the church members would be free to choose how much of their resources to give and never be required to give a set amount of their income unless they wanted to. Also, and just as importantly, there would never be any physical, emotional, or sexual exploitation of any kind.

Joe's therapist asked that he imagine very specific details of this ideal ministry and what it would be like to be a member of such a congregation. These details would include such things as: visualizations of church members participating in the ministry, their emotional expressions, songs, fellowship together, etc. Joe's homework was to meditate on this ideal ministry each night before going to sleep. He was taught how to utilize the five second meditation technique described in Appendix #1. Remarkably, Joe's therapy turned out to be very effective and within just two weeks he began to feel much less anxious and upset about leaving the church. He was even able to share honestly with some of the other church members about his reason for leaving without identifying his female friend. He told them exactly how he felt about what was going on and how he must break away and move on. There were some members of the congregation who tried to convince him not to leave, however, he was not dissuaded and was able to effectively make a clean break from the church. Unfortunately, there was nothing that could be done to shut down the ministry as no other person would come forward charging the minister with sexual misconduct. Due to the tax exempt status of the church, no financial improprieties could be implicated. In order to meet his strong desire to belong to a religious community, Joe was able to join a ministry which was more conventional and did not exploit the members.

Although Joe's experience with a cult was not as dramatic as some, this illustration shows how it is possible to break free when a person realizes how harmful and destructive it is. It can take a great deal of courage and is not an easy thing to do. As stated before, some cult members will never leave for any reason and will cling to their core beliefs even though those beliefs may defy reality. Core beliefs are much like symptoms, they "don't like to be erased or eliminated. They get pissed." (Steve Andreas). There must be an overpowering reason to give them up and be transformed into something more positive. RIT offers this opportunity. Moving on now, let's consider guilt and shame as they relate transforming negative core beliefs.

Toxic Guilt and Shame

Toxic guilt and shame - why would I group these two issues together? I say because they go together like the old song, "Love and Marriage;" they go together like a horse and carriage. Unlike love and marriage and a horse and carriage, however, they are far from being anything positive. Quite the opposite, they can be very destructive when they become negative core beliefs. Often these beliefs start out in early childhood, when a child must decide who is to blame for all of the terrible things happening around them. Children are unable to understand the true nature of the abuse, chaos and dysfunction which they are exposed to. Very often, they make the decision that it is their fault and they are somehow to blame. The human mind was designed in such a way that it must decide on things one way or another even though the decision may be flawed. A good example of this could be Mommy and Daddy always fighting and arguing with one another. Little Joe or Joleen sees this and needs find a resolution in their own mind. We presented this in our first illustration (Illustration #1), when we spoke about negative self-talk and the "it's my fault syndrome." It is extremely common and often leads to the negative core beliefs of and guilt and shame. Once established, other problems may develop such as low self-esteem, people pleasing, anxiety, depression, addictions, and the expression of negative attention in all sorts of ways.

Of course, not all negative core beliefs are the same. Some people can go in an entirely different direction, even to the point of concluding that nothing is ever their fault. This situation often arises when few - if any - limits are placed on children while growing up. This too produces negative behaviors such as selfishness, narcissism, sexual exploitation, lack of boundaries etc., etc. These individuals seem to lack any sense of appropriate feelings of guilt and shame. Their negative core beliefs are completely different. You could even label them an "it's never my fault syndrome." We will be talking about that in a future topic and illustration. Because we are dealing with inappropriate and toxic guilt and shame here, we will only be presenting the following an illustration of Joleen, who developed these problems at a very early age.

Illustration #8

Joleen is a 24 year old young adult raised as an only child in a very dysfunctional family with a great deal of emotional and physical abuse. Her father was alcoholic and her mother was very codependent in her relationship with him. Joleen remembers her mother and father being in a constant state of turmoil, arguing and even physically fighting at times. Because Joleen was unable to understand what was going on, she automatically concluded that it was her fault and that she was to blame (i.e., the "it's my fault syndrome"). She tried to help as much as she could by always trying to please her parents so that they wouldn't fight. She would even try to comfort and provide counseling to her mother when she

35

became upset. In her heart, Joleen had love for both her mother and father and wished that things were different between them. Although her efforts to make things better never worked, she kept trying. Her mother would often ask Joleen for advice, which was very confusing to her. Finally, her father's alcoholism and abuse became so unbearable that her mother left home with Joleen and they went to live with her maternal grandmother. Eventually, Joleen's mother filed for divorce and she rarely saw her father after that.

The guilt and shame that she felt about not being able to help her parents never left her. As time went on, she continued to try to accommodate others and often was not honest and authentic with them. People pleasing became a way of life for her. She felt like she could never really be herself. Whenever anything negative happened in her life, she automatically felt guilty and ashamed. This was especially true when it came to relationships. A major crisis came when she was having problems with her boyfriend who became very demanding and controlling of her. She became so emotionally upset that she began thinking of suicide. She felt guilty and ashamed that she was somehow unable to work things out. The straw that broke the camel's back, however, was when her boyfriend left her. Joleen felt so full of shame and guilt that she attempted suicide by cutting her wrists. Fortunately, her roommate came home and discovered what she had done and called 911. She was taken to the emergency room and then admitted to a nearby psychiatric hospital where she stayed for 2 weeks. After she was deemed safe for discharge, Joleen was referred to an outpatient center for follow-up treatment. Her therapist took Joleen's suicide attempt very seriously and knew from experience that Joleen required a change in perception about how she viewed herself. There were a number of different ways he could have worked on this problem, such as traditional psychodynamic psychotherapy or cognitive behavioral therapy (CBT), but he decided to use radical imagination therapy (RIT) instead. He taught Joleen how to meditate using the 5 second breathing technique (Appendix#1) and asked her about what her ideal self might look like and be like. He was very specific with his questions asking all sorts of questions such as: where she was; how she looked; how others might respond to her in an ideal way; and what her ideal significant others might say to her? The purpose for doing this was not to deny how it really was while growing up but rather to give Joleen a more positive way of thinking how it could have been and what that would have been like. Not stopping there, her therapist instructed Joleen to make up an imaginary story about how that situation could be resolved. He said that the story could be it about anything that her imagination could come up with (i.e., an animal, a real person, a fictional person, a cartoon character, or who or whatever she could imagine).

Joleen did very well with both suggestions. She described her ideal self as being a very confident and courageous young woman who would always speak her mind. She said that when people would try to persuade her to do something that she was uncomfortable doing, she would never give in to them. She said that she would always be very honest with people even though it might hurt their feelings. Joleen's therapist again became very specific with her and asked her give examples of how that would feel like and be like. The example that Joleen gave was when a friend tried to persuade her to sign a petition that she didn't agree with and she saw herself speaking up and presenting her own point of view. Coaching her, her therapist had her describe specific details such as where she was and exactly what she said. Joleen said that before this exercise, she would have felt guilty and ashamed for not giving in to her friend. After this exercise, she said that she felt very confident and courageous about herself. When asked to construct a healing story, Joleen came up with one of her favorites, "The Little Engine That Could." She said that she imagined herself being that little engine, able to pull a heavy load (guilt and shame) up over a steep mountain and overcome it. Her therapist again asked her about the specific details related to this story and about what it felt like when she successfully got to the top of the mountain. Before her bedtime, Joleen was asked to meditate on these two scenarios (i.e., her ideal self and the story about the little engine that could). When he saw her again the following week, Joleen was asked rate her progress on a scale of one to ten, with one being the most improved and ten being the least (Appendix #7). She saw herself as being a two. She said that she was much more confident and comfortable with herself. Joleen was instructed to continue doing her meditations and whenever she felt guilty or ashamed about something to think of these two imaginary scenarios.

Joleen's thoughts and feelings about herself improved
dramatically.

Narcissism, Bullying, Discrimination

Although there are many, many more examples of negative core beliefs that could be presented, we have decided on these three, which are very common: narcissism, bullying, and discrimination. We will be presenting all three of these examples in our final illustration, however, let us first define each, one by one.

Narcissism can best be defined as being self-absorbed with oneself and one's own needs. It usually results from some sort of neglect or even abuse which may very well include overindulgence in childhood. Putting oneself first and even taking advantage of others is often a symptom of narcissism. People with narcissism can often be very manipulative and can even rise to power in organizations of all sorts, and even politics. When mixed with their persuasive qualities and charisma, it is possible for narcissists to influence others in all sorts of negative ways.

Bullying can be defined as targeting another individual or individuals for some kind of personal gain, be it material or psychological. Wikipedia defines bullying as the use of force, coercion, hurtful teasing or threat to abuse, dominate or intimidate. The behavior is often repeated and habitual (Wikipedia).

Discrimination is very much related to both narcissism and bullying. There is a payoff for this individual in that they often get feelings of elation and superiority when they disparage or ridicule a person or group of people for whatever reason. A good definition of discrimination also appears in Wikipedia: "Discrimination is the act of making unjustified distinctions between people based on groups, classes, or other categories to which they belong or are perceived to belong. People may be discriminated on the basis of race, gender, age, religion, disability, or sexual orientation, as well as other categories." (Wikipedia) Discrimination is alive and well in this country and throughout the world and for sure stands out as a negative core belief.

Illustration #9

In this final illustration we have Joe, a 22 year old young adult, who displays all three of the negative core beliefs mentioned above. Joe found himself incarcerated after a very serious road rage incident that resulted in the victim of his rage being seriously injured. The victim, who was Black, could have died but instead was left permanently paralyzed as a result of a spinal cord injury. The incident happened when Joe was inadvertently cut off by the victim while in heavy traffic. Joe became so enraged that he rammed his car into the back of the victim's vehicle, causing the victim to lose control and hit a tree. After this heinous act, Joe continued on his way, however, his license plate number was recorded by another motorist. The police were called and Joe was subsequently arrested. It immediately became a headline in the news and because the victim was Black, racial issues became a major factor as well. Joe was released on bond and a trial date was set. Joe was very adamant that because he was cut off in traffic, his actions were somehow justified. His court appointed attorney did his best to provide a defense for him, however, he was ultimately convicted of criminal intent to do harm while driving and was sentenced to two years in prison.

It was in prison that Joe had a time to reflect on what he had done. About two months into his sentence, he requested to see the prison social worker to help him deal with his remorse related to his negative behavior. He reported having nightmares about the road rage incident as well as about the trial. It seemed clear to the social worker that Joe was ready to process his road rage behavior and deal with his own issues related to it.

 A full psychological assessment was done, and it was found that he had a number of very concerning negative childhood experiences while growing up (Adverse Childhood Experiences, or ACES). He was the oldest of three children in a very physically and emotionally abusive family. His father was alcoholic and he never felt loved by either of his parents. Corporal punishment was the preferred method of discipline. Joe learned from an early age that in order to get attention he had to show off and put other people down. He admitted that he modeled many of his behaviors after his father who was very prejudiced against minorities, especially Blacks. Joe also admitted that he became a bully at school which made him feel like a "real man." Being dominant over others became a way of life for him. Because he was muscular and large in stature, he was very easily able to get by with this without retaliation.

Given his history and feelings of remorse, Joe's social worker decided to use RIT to address his problems. As is the usual case, a major goal of RIT therapy is to achieve a perceptual change which would allow him to think about and even experience his negative actions in a different and more positive way. The therapy was designed not to negate or deny his responsibility, but rather to see how it could have been different.

After getting Joe's approval to move forward with this unusual type of therapy, his therapist decided to utilize two RIT techniques that he felt could be helpful. The first was having him to imagine the act of asking for forgiveness. The second was imagining an ideal outcome regarding the incident. Both of these therapy approaches required that Joe learn to meditate. Because he was unfamiliar with meditation, he was taught the five second breathing technique of meditation (Appendix #1) which he was able to master very quickly.

 In utilizing the first RIT technique, Joe was asked to imagine a scenario of sincerely asking for forgiveness related to his road rage behavior. It was suggested that he visualize this as realistically and sincerely as possible, playing out in front of him much like a movie with all of the verbal and emotional expressions in it. After some initial hesitation, Joe was able to do this successfully. He reported back that his apology was like a burden which was suddenly lifted from his shoulders. He said that he was able to visualize the victim accepting his apology in his "mind's eye," which was very comforting to him. Of course, Joe knew in his heart that this may never happen, however, it comforted him to know that this was the outcome that he hoped for. After this session, Joe was advised to meditate on this scenario each night just before retiring.

During his next therapy session, he reported feeling a little better. On a scale of one to ten, with one being the most improved, he rated himself as a three. The second RIT technique introduced involved imagining a pretended ideal outcome which did not result in either Joe's road rage behavior or the accident. His therapist asked Joe to come up with a scenario in which after being cut off by the driver, he was able to handle the situation in an entirely different manner which was nonviolent. Joe reported that he would just say to himself: "That was a stupid and dangerous thing to do. I hope he never does that again to anyone else. I'm going to get his license plate number and let the police know about his reckless driving." He then used his cell phone to call the police.

 Joe was again asked to meditate on both of these imagined scenarios just before going to sleep. As usual, in his note pad, he was asked to rate his improvement at the end of each day. To his amazement, his ratings were in the ones and twos. He continued his meditations up until he was released from prison for good behavior after a year and a half. At that time he wrote a letter of apology to his victim and asked if someday they might meet together.

Why did these techniques work so well for Joe? I say it all gets back to the same old issue of perceptual change.

The positive imagined outcomes presented made it possible for Joe to see how these negative circumstances and negative core beliefs can be altered. It also showed the wonders of neuroplasticity. The circumstances were altered in such a way that Joe automatically grabbed onto a better solution and outcome than the road rage behavior (Milton H. Erickson) . His overall feelings about the situation demonstrated that. He no longer was a prisoner of his old thoughts and feelings.

Summary

It can never be said loud enough that negative core beliefs are in the "eye of the beholder." To some people they are absolute truths. In this book, however, we have defined them very simply as belief systems which are in some way harmful to the self or to others. Positive core beliefs, on the other hand, promote health and wellbeing to oneself and others. I would hazard to say that, for the most part, positive core beliefs far outnumber the negative ones. Once a core belief system is established, there is a tendency to cling to it and even defend it at all costs.

In considering how negative core beliefs get started, they often result from the influence of a significant person or persons in one's life. This may be parents, peers, and even charismatic leaders of all sorts. There is a strong tendency to adopt the ideologies of these persons even though they may fly in the face of common sense and reality. This can be seen time and time again in cults and other repressive organizations, be they religious or otherwise.

In this book we have discussed a few of the major negative core beliefs that have an influence on our behavior (i.e., negative selftalk, eating disorders, addictions, hoarding, cults, guilt and shame, as well as narcissism, bullying and discrimination). Although there are many different ways to change or transform these negative belief systems, we have chosen RIT as a major treatment modality. Our reason for choosing RIT is based on our knowledge about the power of our imagination. We believe strongly that our imagination shares the same neurology as real memories and that our unconscious mind is influenced by these memories (even though they are just imagined). When we stimulate our mind with a more positive solution, we automatically grab on to that solution and it quickly becomes an unconscious driver of our thoughts and behaviors.

 Doing RIT well requires the utilization of very imaginative creative ideas which promote positive change and healing. The individual or individuals with the problem needs to actively participate in the development of these ideas as well as agree to try them. Acceptance that there is a problem is a key first step in this process. Once this is accomplished change becomes much easier. After the initial step of acceptance, planning, implementation and repetition complete the process of transformation.

In this book you have seen how transforming negative core beliefs can be life changing. I am reminded of our example of the famous rapper Ice-T and how he gave up his criminal activity because he imagined himself doing something different which was very positive. The payoff for doing this literally transformed his life. Our illustration of Joe and his "crusty pizza" was another example of this. We feel strongly that RIT may be a path forward for some of those individuals caught up in our criminal justice system. Of course, acceptance and a willingness to give it a try is a requirement.

It is our belief that the prevention of negative core
beliefs in the first place would be the best path forward.
Numerous studies have shown that early environmental
influences and childhood experiences contribute to them.
ACES, better known as adverse childhood experiences,
have been studied extensively in this regard. They have
been shown to contribute to all sorts of physical and
emotional problems including negative core beliefs.
Nipping them in the bud before they get established
should be a goal of the future. Until then, we will need to
do the best we can to transform them. We feel that the
use of RIT can be an important way to accomplish this.

Appendix

In this appendix we have included a number of important concepts related to transforming negative core beliefs. We have also included some material from our previous books which apply to this process. We will start by illustrating how to induce a meditative state using a five second countdown breathing technique.

1. Get into a quiet and comfortable space where you will not be disturbed. Relax your body, close your eyes, and notice your breathing. Do this until you are completely relaxed from head to toe. Next, with each exhaled breath, visualize each number as you slowly count down from 5 to 1 (i.e., exhale, 5; exhale, 4; exhale, 3; exhale, 2; exhale, 1). A useful technique for visualizing the numbers is to see them in your "mind's eye" as balls of light going from one side of your mind to another as you count down. You can play with this and use all sorts of visualizations or anything else you would like. After getting to the number one, you should be in a very relaxed and meditative state sufficient to employ your self-directed RIT technique. You may notice that your eyelids begin to flutter at this point. This is a normal reaction which many people experience. You are now ready to begin your self-directed RIT technique. Once you have finished your session and are ready for arousal, you can very simply arouse yourself by reversing the breathing process counting up from 1 to 5

(i.e., exhale, 1; exhale, 2; exhale, 3; exhale 4; exhale, 5). At this point, give yourself the suggestion that you are fully awake, alert, and ready to have a wonderful rest of the day. You may want to practice this procedure a few times to get the hang of it.

2. Addictions and even compulsions go hand in hand with negative core beliefs. In controlling them, find something in your life so powerful that you would never violate it. Then link that special something to the solution of your addiction compulsion (i.e., deny God; deny Jesus; deny Buddha; harm your children or spouse; sacrifice your principles; etc., etc.). Write it down. Memorize it. Remind yourself of it each time that the temptation to fall to the addiction or compulsion comes up. You can use this technique on such things as alcohol, drugs, cigarettes, overeating, or anything else. It is important to remember that if for some reason you give in and fall to your addiction or compulsion, you should promise yourself that you will get right back on track. Relapse is probable, however, it is not defeat. Stay the course and get back on that horse that bucked you off.

Now, I would like to give you an example of how Milton Erickson helped an alcoholic patient who came in for help with his alcohol problem. Colonel Joe Jones was a World War II Ace Air

Force pilot who was referred to Dr. Erickson because he was getting himself into trouble with women and when he would drink he would come across, he would put it, "as a lush," and was perceived as being overly aggressive with them. He came to Erickson to help him to figure out how to solve this problem. He brought with him a box full of military medals displaying all of his accomplishments and awards for heroism and showed them to Erickson. Erickson pushed the medals aside and said he didn't give a damn about them. He went on to say that he thought Jones was a coward, one of the biggest cowards that he had ever met. Erickson then asked Jones what he usually drinks at the bar. The Colonel was appalled at Erickson's behavior but said that he usually orders up a double shot of whiskey with a large beer chaser to start. Erickson reiterated that he thought Jones was a coward, and said that his therapy that day was to go out and order up his usual drinks and toast that Bastard Erickson (paradoxical intention). He then told Jones to come back and let him know how that works out for him. Six months later Col. Jones came back clean and sober to thank Erickson for what he had done for him (Milton H. Erickson).

This story illustrates the power that our core beliefs can play in gaining control of a problem. No way was this alcoholic pilot going to be called a coward because of his drinking. Core beliefs are strong and you too can use them in controlling addictions and compulsions.

3. Controlling anxiety can be a big problem for many of us. The following is a healing story which can also relate to transforming negative core beliefs. This story is called "The Anxious Duck." It is possible to use this story with children as well as adults. It is a story which gets in touch with feelings as well as the intensity of anxiety. It also introduces a role model, a turtle, for the anxious duck to emulate and observe. In the story a new choice is offered up as you will see below.

"Once upon a time there was an anxious duck. His heart would race at the slightest sight or sound. He would look up, look down, look right, look left, and then look all around in just that order. He would even get anxious just thinking about what the other ducks might be thinking about him. He did this for a long, long time. One day when he was looking down, who should he see but a turtle lumbering along toward the pond. The turtle was just enjoying the day and looking forward to a nice cool swim and maybe even a juicy water bug to dine on. The anxious duck kept watching this turtle, so calm and carefree, that he forgot to look up, forgot to look down, forgot to look right, forgot to look left, and even forgot to look all around. He didn't even care what the other ducks might be thinking about

him. He just kept his eyes on the turtle, so calm
and carefree. The turtle didn't mind. He just kept
on calmly lumbering along toward the pond.
Suddenly, the anxious duck had a thought. It was
a thought that hadn't occurred to him before.
Why can't I be like that turtle, so calm and
carefree? I can! I can! I can be like that turtle, the
duck thought. It is possible! So the duck started
following the turtle, looking around comfortably
just enjoying the day. Soon they were at the pond
and they both took a swim. The turtle got his
juicy water bug and the duck even caught a little
fish for his dinner."

This story can be read over and over again and
meditated on. It can even be acted out with
children or adults. It has the ability to change
one's perception about anxiety and discover what
is possible in a fun way.

4. Guilt and shame can be very incapacitating,
    especially for those harboring negative core
    beliefs who are unable to make amends for the
    wrongs they have committed or feel they have
    committed. Religiously oriented people can
    imagine themselves in a place (maybe in
    Heaven) sitting before a group of elders
    admitting all of their wrongs, seeking
    forgiveness and redemption. Kindly receive their
    blessings and forgiveness. For others, it may be
    helpful to just imagine asking for sincere
    forgiveness for the wrongs committed.

5. Another very good method in changing the perception of a negative core belief is to imagine yourself in a movie theater watching yourself doing all of the actions associated with that belief (i.e., overeating, hoarding, being a cult member, etc.). Play this movie in black and white. Stop the movie before it ends and then play it backwards to the beginning. Now imagine playing it again in vivid color only doing just the opposite of the actions associated with the negative core belief (i.e., eating in a healthy way, not hoarding, not being a cult member, etc.). This gives our brain a different and more positive focus without ignoring the previous self-defeating negative behaviors. It transforms them.

6. In dealing with the compulsion to over- or undereat, imagine yourself at your ideal weight (not too heavy or not too thin). Meditate on that image every day. You can use the 5 second breathing technique should you desire (Appendix #1). You may be pleasantly surprised at how well this works. It can also work with other addictions and compulsions as well.

7. Keeping a log of your RIT meditations is a very good way of tracking of your progress related to transforming your negative core beliefs. We recommend using a 1 to 10 rating scale with 10 being the least progress and 1 being the most. This record keeping can be very easily done by using any type of notepad or electronic device.

Importantly, this type of self-assessment can also be used for researching the effectiveness of RIT in transforming negative core beliefs.

8. The creation of a Power Anchor can be an extremely effective way to deal with negative core beliefs. Essentially, Power Anchors are triggers which get in touch with the resourceful self or desired outcome. They carry with them all the feelings, sights, sounds, tastes, and even smells of this outcome (the five senses). They are positive solutions embedded in some sort of internal or external symbolic representation, be it a touch, image, sound, etc. It is important to make this symbolic representation positive, otherwise it has the potential to reinforce the problem state. It can represent such things as the ideal family, ideal circumstances, or really anything else which has been problematic. It can represent a vision of anything which triggers a positive response. This may be a castle or mansion with many rooms or anything else which stimulates a positive response.

Favorite Concepts, Quotes, Poems, and Prayers

Much of the following material is taken from our previous books. Some is new.

1. "A lie repeated three times too often becomes some people's reality." (D. Trent Lewis) Favorite Quote

2. "Out of suffering have emerged the strongest of souls; the most massive characters are seared with scars." (Khalil Gibran) Favorite Quote

3. "Go confidently in the direction of your dreams. Live the life that you have imagined." (Henry David Thoreau) Favorite Quote

4. "If human beings could see their thoughts feelings and words go out into the atmosphere up on the ethers and gather more of their kind, they not only would be amazed at what they gave birth to but would also scream for deliverance." (Unveiled Mysteries, Godfrey Ray King) Favorite Quote

5. "Each person is a unique individual. Hence psychotherapy should be formulated to meet the uniqueness of the individual's needs, rather than tailoring the person to the

Procrustean bed of hypothetical theory of human behavior." (Milton H. Erickson) Favorite Concept

6. "Your task is that of altering, not abolishing." (Milton H. Erickson in Rossie and Ryan) Favorite Concept

7. "Nothing happens unless first a dream." Carl Sandburg) Favorite Quote

8. "Radical Imagination Therapy is a form of therapy which uses imagination to heal a variety of psychological wounds. It is based on the neurolinguistics programming presupposition that imagination shares the same neurology as real memories. In applying this presupposition, it is possible to imagine a solution in the 'mind's eye' which then becomes a real solution. It works because our unconscious mind automatically grabs onto it as a better solution than the one we are using." (D. Trent Lewis) Favorite Concept

9. "Symptoms don't like to be erased or eliminated, they get pissed." (Steve Andreas) Favorite Concept

10. "Faith does not permit of telling. It must be lived to be self-propagating." (Mahatma Gandhi) Favorite Quote

11. "Your life is what your thoughts make it." (Author Unknown) Favorite Quote

12. "The power of imagination makes us infinite." (John Muir) Favorite Quote

13. "Life is an adventure, dare it." (Mother Teresa) Favorite Quote

14. "Whatever the mind of man can conceive and believe, it can achieve." (Napoleon Hill) Favorite Quote

15. "Imagination is more important than knowledge." (Albert Einstein) Favorite Quote

16. "Neurons that fire together, wire together." (Neurology Concept) Favorite Concept

17. "When you have bad memories which may be true or may be false, wouldn't it be much better to seek a redemption for yourself or for others and then use those bad memories to build other memories which are much better and serve a good purpose." (D. Trent Lewis) Favorite Quote

18. "Imagination shares the same neurology as real memories." (NLP presupposition) Favorite Concept

19. "Allow the unconscious to do the work." (Milton H. Erickson) Favorite Concept

20. "I had to clear up my idea that I was a worthless person. Because until I did, I acted like I was a worthless person. I did things that were self-destructive to confirm that I was a worthless person. I am so glad that I believe that I am really okay." (D. Trent Lewis) Favorite Quote

21. "Suppose that you woke up one morning and there was a miracle and all of your problems were solved. Tell me all about that." (Steve deShazer) Favorite Concept

22. "The therapeutic procedures or techniques utilized must be congruent with your client's thoughts, feelings and verbalizations otherwise those procedures will not be acceptable consciously or unconsciously and change will be inhibited. Clients will resist your best efforts to help them change." (D. Trent Lewis) Favorite Concept

23. "If you look deep enough into any behavior, no matter how dysfunctional, you will most usually find a positive intention in there some place." (Virginia Satir) Favorite Concept

24. "Each individual has their own map of the world. It is not the map that limits people but rather the choices that they feel that they have available." (NLP Presupposition, Dilts, Bandler) Favorite Concept

25. "Please tell me about all of the positive things that you have learned by having your problems?" (Steve deShazer) Favorite concept

26. "When you are able to perceive your problems in a different and more positive way, which is agreeable to you, you will find yourself getting better and better." (D. Trent Lewis) Favorite Concept

27. "It has been shown that it is possible to write over bad memories and experiences and also inject new content into those memories." (November 2009 Issue of Discover Magazine) Favorite Concept

28. "Visiting the land of how it could have been creates positive feelings, visions, and possibilities for future changes." (D. Trent Lewis) Favorite Quote

29. "Language, Loops, and Portals to Change: As our thoughts (real or imagined) are put into words and behaviors, messages are conveyed which develop into patterns and loops. As these patterns get established and internalized, they develop a life of their own. Language which is either verbal or nonverbal, carries connotations and even expectations for either positive or negative change." (D. Trent Lewis) Favorite Concept

30. "Life is but a thought." (Sara Teasdale) Favorite Quote

31. "He who has a why to live can bear almost any how." (Friedrich Nietzsche) Favorite Quote

32. "Only a life lived for others is a life worthwhile." (Albert Einstein) Favorite Quote

33. "If you spend your whole life waiting for the storm, you'll never enjoy the sunshine." (Morris West) Favorite Quote

34. "The power of imagination makes us infinite." (John Muir) Favorite Quote

35. "Dreams are the ultimate in imaginative thinking. They are innovative ways of finding a solution to our inner struggles and can be used as portals to emotional healing." (D. Trent Lewis) Favorite Concept

36. "Any therapy should always be done in accordance with the needs of the patient, whatever they may be, and not based in any way on arbitrary classifications. Psychologically oriented forms of therapy properly employed need always be in relationship to the patient's capacity to receive and understand." (Milton H. Erickson) Favorite Quote

37. "Positive personal change can be attained when changing the context of where a problem occurs, the internal mental processes, the internal state, or the external behavior of the person." (NLP Concept for Change) Favorite Concept

38. "Imagine what you want. Discover what you wished for." (Author Unknown) Favorite Quote

39. "Everything is energy and that's all there is to it. Match the frequency of the reality you want and you cannot help but get that reality. It can be no other way. This is not philosophy. This is physics." (Albert Einstein) Favorite Quote

40. "Feelings that are expressed will limit themselves." (Author Unknown) Favorite Quote

41. "Whatever you are, be a good one." (Abraham Lincoln)

42. Isabell's Prayer: "Oh precious Holy Spirit, beloved of our souls, we adore you. Guide us, strengthen us, enlighten us, and console us. Tell us what we should do. Give us your orders. We promise to submit ourselves to all that you desire of us and to accept all that you permit to happen to us. Let us know only your will." (Isabelle Robertson) Prayer

References

Andreas, S. (2012) Transforming Negative Self-Talk: Practical Effective Exercises-1st ed. New York, NY., Norton & Company, Inc.

Andreas, S., Andreas, C., (1987) Change Your Mind and Keep the Change-Printing 4, 5, 6, 05, 04, Moab, UT,. 84532 Real People Press

Andreas S., Andreas, C., (1989) Heart and Mind, Real People Press, Bolder Co., 80302

Andreas, A., (2002) Transforming Yourself, Real People Press, Bolder, Co., 80302

Andreas, S., Faulkner, Charles, Editors, (1996) N.L.P., The New Technology Achievement, William Morrow Paperback, Harper Collins Publishers NY., NY., 10007

Andreas, S. (20006) Six Blind Elephants: Understanding Ourselves and Others, Real People Press, Bolder, Co., 80302

Andreas, S., Andreas, C., Damara (1994) Core Transformation: Reaching the Wellspring Within, Real People Press, Bolder, Co., 80302

Bandler, Richard, Grinder, John (1970) Frogs into Princes Real People Press, Bolder, Co., 80302

Bandler, Richard, Grinder, John (1982) Reframing, Real People Press, Bolder, Co., 80302

Bradshaw, John (1988 Revised Edition 2005) Healing the Shame that Binds You, Expanded and updated ed. P. cm. Publisher: Health Communications, Inc., 3201 S.W., 15th Street Dearfield Beach, FL. 334422-8190 ISBN 13:978-0-7573-0323-4 ISBN 10:0-0323-4

DeShazer, Steve, Dolan, Yvonne, Berg, Insoo, Kim, Corman, Harry, McCollum, Trapper, Terry (2007 More Than Miracles: The State of the Art of Solution Focused Therapy, Publishers: Routledge Taylor and Francis Group; Hawthorn Press, Inc. New York and London

Erickson, Milton H. (1958) Naturalistic Techniques of Hypnosis---American Society of Clinical Hypnosis---Editor 32 West Cyprus St., Phoenix, Arizona

Erickson, Milton H. (1982) Erickson Approaches to Hypnosis and Psychotherapy Editor Zeig, Jeffrey K., The Milton Erickson Foundation, Brunner/Mazel Publishers New York, New York

Haley, Jay (1993) Uncommon Therapy: The Psychotherapy Techniques of Milton Erickson, W. W. Norton and Company, 500 5th Avenue, N.Y., N.Y.

Jung, C. J., (1986) Memories, Dreams, Reflections Vintage Press, New York, N.Y.

Kelly-Gangie, Carol---Editor (2006) Mother Teresa: Her Essential Wisdom, Fall River Press 122 5th Ave., New York, N.Y. 10011

King, Godfrey Ray (1982) Unveiled Mysteries---Saint Germaine Series., Saint Germaine Press., Schaumburg, Illinois

Lewis, D. Trent and Damsel, Laurel B. (2018) The Principles and Methods of Radical Imagination Therapy, Amazon Books, (Independently Published), ISBN 9781980864813

Lewis, D. Trent and Damsel, Laurel B. (2020) A Self Help Guide to Radical Imagination Therapy, Amazon Books, (Independently Published), KDP, ISBN 9798637270651

Lewis, D. Trent and Damsel, Laurel B. (2022) Healing from Post- Traumatic Stress Injury Using Radical Imagination Therapy, Amazon Books, (Independently Published), KDP, ISBN 9798804164691

Parragon Books (2011) Daily Devotions, Parragon Publications Queen Street House 4 Queen Street Bath BA1 1HE, UK ISBN 978-1-4454-3841-4

Pessio, Albert (1961) Making New Memories, New York University Press, New York, N.Y.

Satir, Virginia (1999) Patterns of Her Magic, Introduction by Steve Andreas, Real People Press, Boulder, Co. 80302

Wikipedia (2022) Anorexia Nervosa, Definition/Prevalence, Authors Credited

Wikipedia (2022) Compulsive Hoarding, Definition/Prevalence, Authors Credited

Wikipedia (2022) Bullying, Definition, Authors Credited

Wikipedia (2022) Discrimination, Definition, Authors Credited

Index

Other books by D. Trent Lewis and Laurel B. Damsel

Lewis, D. Trent and Damsel, Laurel B., (2018) The Principles and Methods of Radical Imagination Therapy, Amazon Books, (Independently Published), KDP, ISBN 9781980864813

Lewis, D. Trent and Damsel, Laurel B. (2020) A Self Help Guide To Radical Imagination Therapy, Amazon Books, (Independently Published), KDP, ISBN 9798637270651

Lewis, D. Trent and Damsel, Laurel B. (2022) Healing from Post- Traumatic Stress Injury Using Radical Imagination Therapy, Amazon Books, (Independently Published), KDP, ISBN 9798804164691

www.ingramcontent.com/pod-product-compliance
Lightning Source LLC
Chambersburg PA
CBHW061301250726
48653CB00002B/719